Supplements

Top 10 Supplements for Men

By
Bring on Fitness

About Bring On Fitness

Our passion for fitness gave life to **Bring On Fitness**. We started with the goal of helping as many people as we can. To educate, motivate and to help change peoples lives for the better. Bring On Fitness is not only for the fitness enthusiasts, but also for the beginner. We strongly believe nothing is more important than learning the basics and creating a strong foundation in both nutrition - through meal planning, and in exercise - by following a specific plan. This is just as important for the beginner, as it is for the experienced athlete.

We set high standards for ourselves, the information we share, and the products we carry. Our goal is to provide you with exceptional products that suit your needs and the knowledge and motivation to help you work towards and achieve your health and fitness goals.

Check us out at www.bringonfitness.com

"Our Mission is to have a positive impact in changing peoples lives. We will deliver the best possible fitness and nutrition solutions that will empower people to achieve their health and fitness goals."

Table of Contents

Introduction **11**

1) Whey Protein.. **13**

Helps in shedding fat and preserves muscle 13

Increases strength and size 13

Reduces hunger 14

Manages stress..14

Improves immunity 15

2) Creatine **16**

Enhances recovery and aerobic performance...................16

Increases bone density...17

Improves brain performance 17

Reduces oxidative stress 17

Protects against traumatic brain injury 18

3) Fish Oil **19**

Helps burn fat 19

Enhances muscle growth..20

Encourages healthy joints 20

Increases energy levels...20

4) Carnitine..**22**

Enhances athletic performance 22

Facilitates faster muscle recovery 22

Improves cardiovascular health 23

5) Casein **24**

Lasts in your system for a longer duration 24

Yields greater gains 25

Helps in enhancing your metabolic rate 25

Yields greater strength 25

Beefs up your teeth 26

6) Glutamine **27**

Beats muscle fatigue 27

Protects from muscle breakdown 28

Boosts your overall health 28

7) Multivitamin/Mineral Supplements **29**

Vitamin A 29

Magnesium 30

Selenium 30

Zinc 30

Copper 31

Vitamin D 31

8) BCAA **32**

Improves muscle protein synthesis *32*

Enhances performance and reduces fatigue *32*

Decreases Muscle Soreness *33*

9) Arginine **34**

10) Beta-Alanine **36**

Improves athletic performance *36*

Increases muscle mass *36*

Improves cognitive function under stress *37*

Conclusion **39**

Sources **41**

Introduction

I want to thank you for choosing this book, *"Supplements - Top 10 Supplements for Men."*

If you have recently turned into a gym rat, you may constantly be on the hunt for the perfect supplement, which will enhance your performance. Every time you hit the gym, you may be tempted to buy all those shiny tubs of mysterious supplements placed on the counter. You may be secretly hoping that it turns you into the vintage Schwarzenegger overnight. No, we are not here to crush your dreams, but loading up on a few generic supplements isn't going to get you the results you are dreaming of.

Just because they are popular doesn't mean they will work for you. Regardless of whether you are an athlete or someone who is trying to build a physique, it's important to know your specific needs and then address them first.

Are you a cyclist? Are you a bodybuilder? Are you a pro power lifter? Are you a marathoner? See, these are the questions you need to ask yourself before you make your pick. When you start with the fundamentals, you can't go wrong. If you are an average guy, you don't need to load up on too many supplements, but some selective supplementation can work wonders for you.

In this book, we have presented you with the top 10 supplements that can give you the results you need. We know how misguided people are when it comes to supplements. For this reason, we wanted to come up with a guide that can show you the right path to supplementation. For anyone who is constantly wondering "Are supplements right for my age?" or

"Will these work for me?" this book should be able to clarify all your doubts.

It's not that you can't function without supplementation, but the lack of it can cause you to feel fatigued and experience serious muscle loss that, in turn, can pave the way for some chronic illnesses. Supplements can be the magic potion you are looking for, but only if you pick the right ones and take them as per the recommended dosage.

1) Whey Protein

When you think of whey protein, you immediately assume that it's meant for large-bodied muscle heads. Now, we aren't entirely refuting this statement if you are doing intense workouts and consuming a diet that is rich in protein, fruit, vitamin-rich veggies with fiber, and high-quality carbs and are still not gaining muscle, whey protein can be a lifesaver. However, that's not the only reason why you should make whey protein a regular feature in your daily routine. Here are a few reasons why whey is good for men.

Helps in shedding fat and preserves muscle

If your original plan was to lose all the excess fat, but you ended up losing a lot of muscle on the way, you seriously need to consider adding whey protein to your diet. It may be interesting to know that as per a 12-week research study conducted in Minnesota, the daily calorie intake of participants was reduced by 500 calories. Of all the participants, some were made to drink an isocaloric mix beverage while others were offered whey. The ones who consumed whey ended up losing about 6.1 percent of their total body fat while preserving better muscles as compared to the other beverage.

Increases strength and size

Have you been struggling to make strength gains? According to a particular study conducted at Baylor University in Waco, Texas, about 19 participants were made to perform resistance training over a period of 10 weeks. They were given 6 g of free amino acids and 14 g of whey casein protein, and the others were given 20 g of placebo. The ones who consumed whey experienced an increase in fat-free mass along with muscle strength. It is highly recommended that you drink whey shake at least an hour prior and post your exercises.

Reduces hunger

Can't seem to get you hunger pangs under control? It's time to try some whey protein. Muscle soreness due to intense workout sessions isn't the only struggle you face while trying to gain muscles and enhance your strength. Being able to get those occasional hunger pangs under control seems like an uphill task for many. It has been observed that people who consume a shake containing 50 g of whey experience reduction in ghrelin (a hormone that triggers hunger), thereby alleviating their hunger pangs. So instead of indulging in an unhealthy snack at the party, try drinking a whey protein shake beforehand.

Manages stress

If you are vulnerable to stress, we may have found the perfect solution for you. A lot of people resort to alcohol to drown their worries but end up feeling even more depressed once the initial high wanes. There are several types of research that show that people who consume whey when they are stressed have reported to be in a better mood for the rest of the day than those who did not. It was concluded that the changes in the brain were made by serotonin and was likely the cause of their upbeat mood.

Improves immunity

A lot of men who haven't exercised in their lives suddenly start performing intense workouts without checking their immunity levels as a result of which most of them start experiencing a reduction in their glutathione levels, which can impact their immune, gastrointestinal, and nervous systems. Reports suggest that consuming whey protein can help these men experience a comparatively minor reduction in their glutathione levels.

2) Creatine

Over the last couple of decades, creatine has been a supplement of choice among professional and recreational athletes and continued to stay in demand. While its popularity has been on a constant rise, a lot of men avoid creatine because of the fear of bulking up too much, but that's a mistake!

Several researchers have suggested that it does a lot more than merely build up your strength and muscle. Not a lot of people know this, but creatine can have a positive impact on a person's memory, bone mineral density, and even reduces oxidative stress. There are so many benefits to consuming creatine on a regular basis that you just shouldn't miss out on. Some of these benefits are mentioned below. Take a look.

Enhances recovery and aerobic performance

Creatine is not only meant for professional endurance athletes but is also crucial for any man who is into rigorous workouts. It has been proven time and again that consuming creatine before prolonged exercise can enhance glycogen stores. Creatine is also helpful in maintaining hydration status and body temperature when exercising in scorching temperatures. Overall, creatine works wonder for athletes as well as non-athletes who are into strenuous workouts.

Increases bone density

Across the globe, osteoporosis, which causes a loss of bone density, has been causing over 8.9 million fractures every year. These cases have been increasing at an alarming rate, and it's about time we started consuming creatine to enhance our bone density. Creatine supplementation has proven to result in a significant increase in the bone mineral content of men as compared with resistance training only. Your bone health may not matter much to you right now, but building strong and healthy bones by consuming creatine can help you prevent osteoporosis as you grow older.

Improves brain performance

Finding it hard to believe? Take it from us that regular consumption of creatine can significantly increase your oxygen utilization capacity in the brain and reduce mental fatigue. Consuming creatine supplementation for six weeks in a row is known to increase the creatine levels in your brain by about 9 percent, and this translates into brainpower!

Reduces oxidative stress

Endurance athletes aren't the only people who suffer from oxidative stress caused by intense training, but anyone who follows an intense training regime is likely to experience it at some point in time. Combine it with incorrect recovery strategies, and you have an absolute recipe for disaster. Several studies have proven the antioxidant effects of creatine and how it promotes better recovery.

Protects against traumatic brain injury

If there's one area where creatine stands out, it has to be its ability to protect you from brain injury. Studies conducted on children as well as adolescents at the university hospital of Heraklion in Greece have shown that creatine consumption after a traumatic brain injury significantly helped in communication as well as recovery time. It also reduces the symptoms of fatigue, dizziness, and numerous headaches.

3) Fish Oil

Contrary to popular belief, fish oil isn't only meant for beautification purposes. Over the years, we have heard a lot about how fish oil can give us nice hair and skin, but there's a lot more to these magic pills than you know. Fish oil is a supplement that everyone should be consuming at some point of time in their lives, especially men who are looking at enhancing their training capacity or building a physique. So why fish oil, you ask? Why can't just eating fish be enough? Well, for one, most of the fish we eat is poorly bred, and secondly, because they contain heavy metals and don't contain enough DHA and EPA, which are needed to reap the optimum benefits of this superfood.

For those of you who are wondering whether fish oil is of any use in building muscles, the answer is a definite "Yes." Here's how it works. Fish oil helps in reducing your cortisol (stress) levels, thereby helping you reduce the total fat percentage in your body. Don't get me wrong; you will still need regular workouts and a balanced diet to achieve this fat loss, but fish oil supplements can shorten your journey to Gainesville. So how exactly does fish oil supplement help us in building the desired physique? Here's how.

Helps burn fat

We all know that bodybuilding and body fat don't go together. The very basis of bodybuilding is to shed fat while gaining muscle; this is why fish oil supplements are ideal. Fish oil supplements do contain fat but not the harmful kinds. It is full of healthy fats, which when consumed, do not get stored in the body as body fat. Instead, it's used as a primary source of energy, thereby increasing metabolic levels and eventually helping us burn more calories, which are stored in our bodies in the form of fat.

Enhances muscle growth

You may think all of these supplements help in building muscles, so what's special about fish oil supplements? The reason why fish oil stands out is due to its ability to reduce the level of stress hormones in your body in no time. Fish oil is also useful in increasing protein synthesis, which in turn helps post-workout muscle recovery while muscle proteins are synthesized by the body.

Encourages healthy joints

If there's one thing that fish oil is popular for, it is for its ability to promote healthy joints by lubricating them, thus preventing muscle soreness, and it aids in fighting conditions like arthritis. Most bodybuilders' joints are largely affected when they build muscles because larger muscles mean they turn so much heavier. The first body part that gets affected is the knees; the regular consumption of fish oil supplements can help prevent this condition.

Increases energy levels

Let's accept that when you are working hard to build your physique, it going to be extremely tiring, both mentally and physically. Intense workouts mean more weights, more volume, less recovery, more reps, and as a result, greater exhaustion. Fish oil supplements can substantially increase your energy levels, boost your metabolism, and offer you the desired results without much struggle.

4) Carnitine

Carnitine supplement has slowly made its way toward popularity as a highly effective pre-workout supplement. Although this supplement has been in existence since the 1980s, it is only recently that it gained acknowledgment in the current market. Even though fancy pre-workout drinks or the so-called fat-burner coffees often replace Carnitine, it doesn't lose its appeal one bit. If you haven't tried this supplement yet, let me give you some reasons that prove that it's worth a try.

Enhances athletic performance

Carnitine can go a long way in helping you build muscle mass. It also increases your energy levels and, in turn, aids in preserving the muscle glycogen reserves. When you are doing high-intensity workouts, carnitine helps in eliminating the lactic acid build up in your muscles within no time. This also means that you will experience minor discomfort during training while increasing your capacity for high-intensity exercises.

Facilitates faster muscle recovery

What's special about carnitine is that it aids in accelerating the short-term as well as long-term recovery of the body. It lends the muscle fibers the capacity to recuperate within a shorter time, especially after your workout sessions. Moreover, carnitine has an uncanny ability to increase free testosterone utilization, which aids in muscle fiber recovery after an intense workout session.

Improves cardiovascular health

Carnitine can easily break down long-chain fatty acids, which help in enhancing your cardiovascular health and boosts up your metabolic rate. Several studies have shown that carnitine supplements can drastically decrease the chances of developing arteriosclerosis. Not only that, but it also eliminates the bad cholesterol from the body, thereby unclogging your arteries.

5) Casein

If you wish to bring out your body's maximum efficiency, there's one thing you shouldn't be taking for granted, and that's high-quality protein. Most of you who have been working out for a long time know that casein is an ideal pre- and post-exercise protein choice. Complete physique transformation requires you to build new muscles while preserving them from "catabolism," which is a muscle stealer. Casein is highly effective in preventing catabolism and helps you reach your goals easily. Casein is a protein derived from milk and mostly found in an Indian food called "Paneer (cottage cheese)." Casein, as a form of protein, is found in larger quantities in milk as compared to whey. Casein is also known to be a slow-digesting protein, which releases slowly in the body, but does this make it any less effective? Absolutely not! In fact, casein is used to build lean muscle mass within a shorter duration.

Here are a few more reasons to love casein:

Lasts in your system for a longer duration

All protein is not created equally. So whether it's egg, soy, animal, whey, or casein protein, all of them have their special benefits. The greatest strength of casein is timing. Casein can offer a slow but steady supply of amino acids, which can last for hours. Don't expect to build your muscles overnight, but a glass of casein-rich milk before you hit the bed would help you build them faster.

Yields greater gains

Wish to build massive muscles instantly? Casein can help you reach your desired goal more quickly. Based on a Texas-based research, in which 36 males performing intense resistance training participated, those who consumed casein in combination with whey yielded a significant and lean muscle mass as compared with other protein supplements. There is no need to stick to a single form of protein when a combo can yield better results.

Helps in enhancing your metabolic rate

If your final goal is fat loss and muscle growth, then casein is your best bet. According to a research conducted in the Netherlands, it was shown that if you multiply casein consumption by two and half times, the male participants experienced a severe boost in their metabolic rate; they could sleep better and had an overall fat balance. It was also reported that the satiety levels of these participants were almost 33 percent higher. In short, casein intake will not only ensure that you lose fat but will also leave you feeling fuller.

Yields greater strength

If you ask people what their workout goals are, they will immediately reply with increased strength as their top priority. A lot of them want to take the shorter route and resort to almost every combination of protein supplements available in the market, only to gain results. According to a Massachusetts study, casein consumption had almost double the impact of other proteins on their chest, leg, and shoulder strength.

Researchers are of the opinion that the credit should go to the anti-catabolic abilities of casein. So the next time you find yourself craving for a late night snack, have a casein shake.

26

Beefs up your teeth

Don't you hate visiting the dentist? Doesn't the very thought of sitting on that dental chair and going through painful procedures make you cringe? According to research conducted in the United Kingdom, casein could be a great way to avoid expensive and painful dental treatments. It was found that casein could protect your teeth from enamel erosion. This is good news for people who can't get rid of the habit of sipping on soft drinks; your casein intake will save your teeth from erosion.

6) Glutamine

L Glutamine is known to be the third most popular bodybuilding supplement across the world. Athletes and bodybuilders regularly use it for recovery and for enhancing their performance. Your body requires large amounts of this protein, especially if you are big on gaining muscles. Commonly, Glutamine is used to achieve the following benefits:

- Fat burning
- Muscle building
- Faster weight loss

While those are the benefits most people look for, science has proven that Glutamine supplement intake has several benefits, including improvement of the brain and digestive health, boost in athletic performance, treatment of a leaky gut, and enhancement of your overall health. Glutamine can be found both in plants and animals. However, you may not get enough Glutamine through your food alone. This is why Glutamine supplements are necessary. They are a great way to boost your immune system while increasing your body's disease-fighting capacity.

Here's why Glutamine should be an essential part of your daily supplementation.

Beats muscle fatigue

Those lactic acid build-ups due to high-intensity training can take a serious toll on your muscles and result in muscle fatigue. According to research conducted by the Louisiana

State University School of Medicine, Glutamine can help to battle this effect. The researchers found that participants who consumed 2 g of glutamine showed elevated bicarbonate blood levels about 90 minutes post intake. This can help to reduce the "burn" caused by lactic acid accumulation. It is also vital to know that protein intake can get accelerated when faced with acidic conditions, thereby impeding muscle catabolism.

Protects from muscle breakdown

Skeletal muscle is the main reservoir of glutamine, and any prolonged shortcomings in this area can result in considerable loss of muscle mass. Reduction in plasma glutamine levels in response to workouts can lead to catabolism to supply free glutamine to the immune system as well as other parts of the body. Thus, glutamine supplements can offer your muscle cells a supply, which is not necessarily extracted from the skeletal muscle, thereby preventing muscle breakdown.

Boosts your overall health

Glutamine's primary function is to supply fuel to the immune cells so they can fight all sorts of infections. Glutamine supplementation can also help in situations where high-intensity training results in the depletion of your body's overall Glutamine levels. It also helps in reducing the risk of neutrophil destruction induced by exercise while eliminating infection-triggering foreign invaders.

7) Multivitamin/Mineral Supplements

Regardless of how religiously you are following a particular diet, how dedicated you are to nutrition, or how rich in variety your meals are, if you want to be an ace athlete, you will need a multivitamin/mineral supplement.

Our bodies are good at absorbing all the micronutrients we are fed, but as we keep performing intense workouts, these micronutrients get exhausted pretty quickly. This is why we require multivitamin supplements. These supplements contain doses that are much higher than you can consume in a single day. Using this supplement ensures that you are always in surplus for your requirements and have more than enough to sustain the energy levels for your overall health.

We highly recommended taking these multivitamins supplements twice a day for better results. That said, you should consult a medical practitioner before you take any supplement.

Vitamin A

Vitamin A is also referred to as retinol and is mainly found in eggs, fish, milk, yogurt, and fortified margarine. This vitamin can perform several functions, including maintaining the health of your skin, eyesight, immune system, and the mucous lining of your nose. Typically, men require about 0.7 mg per day, but if you are an athlete or into intense exercise, this dosage will go up.

Magnesium

Magnesium can be obtained from various food sources, such as meat, fish, leafy vegetables, bread, and even dairy food. It can help to convert the food we consume into energy, and it helps us maintain our bone health. The recommended dose for men is 300 mg per day, but if you have an underlying medical condition, this dose may vary. Again, consult your medical practitioner before you take a magnesium supplement.

Selenium

Selenium is full of antioxidants that protect your cells from any damage. Several types of research even suggest that selenium supplements can help to reduce the likelihood of prostate cancer. Another study by the American Medical Association concluded that selenium or vitamin E supplements, in combination or alone in specific doses, could be highly effective against prostate and other cancers. The recommended dose of selenium for men is 0.75 mg each day.

Zinc

Zinc helps our bodies to process all the fat, protein, and carbohydrate we get from our food. It is also highly effective in wound healing. Men require about 5.5 to 9.5 mg of zinc supplements per day depending upon your exercise routine.

Copper

Copper is found in nuts, shellfish, and offal, but your body isn't always capable of absorbing the fiber from the food you eat. Copper supplements can benefit you to a large extent in this context. One of the primary functions of copper is producing white and red blood cells, thereby boosting your immunity and keeping you from feeling exhausted. Men can take about 1.2 mg of copper each day.

Vitamin D

We all know that vitamin D can be gained from exposure to the sun, but most adults can't afford this due to their busy lifestyle and so they need a vitamin D supplement. Foods that contain vitamin D are fish, some breakfast cereals, and spreads.

8) BCAA

A commonly asked question is whether or not BCAA supplementation is required for the general population as well as athletes or bodybuilders. The answer is certainly as "yes," but it's only when you experience the power of these supplements that you will be completely convinced. BCAAs are nothing but metabolites that denote lean mass for the young as well as middle-aged population. BCAAs make up about 35 percent of the overall muscle tissue, so the more your body uses them for energy, the more they will slow down the breakdown of muscle cells and reduce muscle loss in men.

Let's look at some of its benefits.

Improves muscle protein synthesis

BCAAs are famous for kick-starting protein synthesis. Along with BCAAs, aspartate, alanine, and even glutamate are taken into muscle tissue for generating energy. It is aimed for muscle to burn BCAAs for energy while working out, making it essential for your performance. Given that BCAAs can be extremely beneficial to trigger protein synthesis, the lean muscle tissue reserve can keep your metabolism going.

Enhances performance and reduces fatigue

BCAAs perform most impressively in enhancing endurance performance and reducing fatigue. Burning BCAAs as energy maintains the ATP energy levels when you perform glycogen-depleting workouts. A study showed that participants who ingested 300 mg of BCAAs per day and later on completed an intense exercise trial exhibited as much as 17.2 percent resistance to fatigue than placebo.

Decreases Muscle Soreness

There have been several studies on trained as well as untrained participants that prove that BCAAs can be extremely useful in reducing muscle soreness and allowing faster recuperation. Researchers believe that the success of BCAAs lies in their ability to supply enough amino acids. BCAAs can be a gem of a workout supplement as they are perfectly capable of preserving muscle fibers, reducing soreness, and encouraging you to work out at a higher intensity.

Some more reasons why endurance athletes prefer BCAAs are as follows:

- Promotes fat burning
- Equalizes muscle build up between the old and young
- Prevents muscles loss
- Improves insulin health and diabetes risk

9) Arginine

L-arginine is a vital amino acid found in the human diet. Given its interactions with a molecule known as the nitric oxide, arginine is used in dietary supplementation. This gas resides in your blood vessels for a short time and helps to improve blood flow while arginine enhances synthesis.

L-arginine is known to be the first nitric oxide booster that has been studied in depth. As soon as people realized its effectiveness, arginine started to be sold as a dietary supplement. Arginine works through the stimulation of the NOS enzyme, especially the variant that is found in blood vessels, with the help of a receptor known as the alpha-2 adrenergic receptor.

If you choose the L-arginine supplement, you can expect the below changes to occur:

- A 5 g dosage of arginine before your workout session can enhance your performance, especially as regards anaerobic endurance.
- The efficacy of arginine is entirely dependent upon the state of one's intestines. What you consumed before the workout session can also make a large difference in determining how effective arginine will be.

Here are about 10 reasons why you should be ingesting an arginine supplement:

- As we age, our arteries can get blocked due to fat, sodium, and cholesterol. Arginine and nitric oxide help in relaxing the blood vessels and eliminate plaque buildup, thereby lowering blood pressure and reducing the chances of heart stroke.

- Arginine works wonders by lowering your bad cholesterol levels and increasing the good cholesterol in your body.
- A lesser-known benefit of arginine is that it aids in boosting your energy levels while increasing blood flow and oxygen that rushes to your heart, brain, and muscles.
- Most athletes and bodybuilders consume arginine because of its ability to increase muscle endurance.
- The main function of your kidneys is to filter your blood of toxins that are excreted through urine. According to several studies, arginine has been found to help the kidneys function more efficiently.
- Men over 50 can experience a huge drop in their libido and, as a result, suffer from erectile dysfunction or other sexual problems. Arginine can alleviate most of these problems.
- When your body's hormonal growth slows down, it automatically slows down the muscle growth, too, making you fragile and leaving you exhausted. Arginine supplements can support your hormonal growth and eliminates related issues.

10) Beta-Alanine

Beta-alanine is commonly referred to as the "new creatine." While it doesn't replace the powers of creatine, it brings with it a unique set of abilities. What is beta alanine? It's nothing but a naturally occurring amino acid. It is known to enhance the carnosine levels in skeletal muscle. Beta-alanine offers you the required flexibility needed for an intense workout session. The highest quality beta alanine is found in BULK POWDERS supplement.

Improves athletic performance

Beta-alanine is known to enhance resistance-training performance for bodybuilders and athletes who perform in team sports. A six-week study was conducted on 15 male water polo players. It was found that after consuming 6.4 g of beta-alanine, these players showed a significant improvement in their performance.

Increases muscle mass

This should have been an obvious guess. Beta-alanine can not only increase your muscle mass but can also prevent you from feeling fatigued. A study on beta-alanine showed that it helped in considerably reducing the acid build-up among athletes during high-intensity anaerobic training, which in turn delayed fatigue.

Improves cognitive function under stress

A 30-day study conducted on 18 elite soldiers showed that beta-alanine consumption resulted in enhanced cognitive function during their combat practice. If that wasn't enough, beta-alanine is also highly effective in muscle recovery under stressful circumstances. Some of the other benefits of beta-alanine are as follows:

- Fights aging
- Prevents the development of tumors
- Helps in recovery from brain injury
- Delays fatigue and reduces lactic acid build up

Conclusion

I wish to thank you once again for purchasing this book.

The most significant paradox in our lives today is that we are overfed but still undernourished. Blame it on our lifestyles or the food quality; we are always low on nourishment. Supplementation has become a need for many to achieve the maximum level of critical nutrients in the body. If you happen to be a professional athlete or are into bodybuilding, it has become all the more important to take supplements.

I sincerely hope that this guide was able to shed some light on the exact information you were looking for when it comes to supplementation for men.

Thank you, and remember to share how well these supplement tips work for you. You can do that by writing a review in your Amazon account under Your Orders.

Thank you,

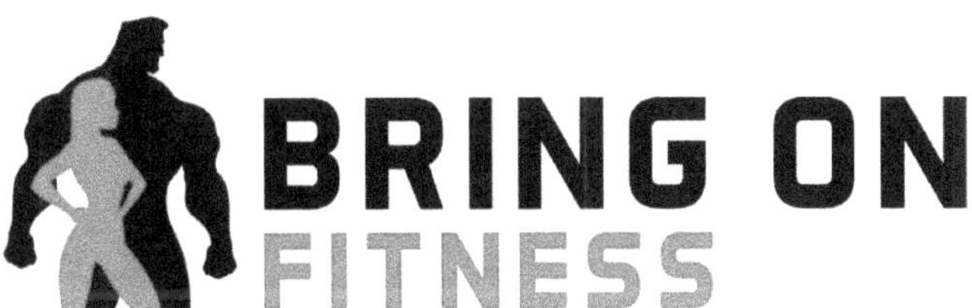

Sources

https://www.selfhacked.com/blog/beta-alanine/

http://l-arginine.com/10-reasons-to-take-l-arginine/

http://main.poliquingroup.com/articlesmultimedia/articles/article/1088/ten_benefits_of_bcaas.aspx

https://www.muscleandperformance.com/supplements-performance/5-reasons-to-take-glutamine

https://www.webmd.boots.com/men/guide/vitamin-mineral-supplements-men

https://www.mensjournal.com/food-drink/5-benefits-of-casein-protein/